Counting Calories For Novice

The Complete Beginner's Flexible Calorie Counting Diet Guide to Enable You Eat the Kind of Food You Love, If It Fits Your Macros and Still Build Muscle, Lose Weight and Burn Fat

Laura Campbell

TABLE OF CONTENT

CHAPTER ONE

LETS CONTROL YOUR DIET WITH THIS FOLLOWING STEPS

Essential to weight reduction and long-term weight control is understanding whilst you're hungry, what to devour for that starvation, and when to stop eating after you sense complete. To assist my customers with this assignment, I created a smooth tool I call "appestat" — an urge for food thermostat — to explain the body's hunger and fullness cues. Mastering the way to study your "appestat" will give you new knowledge of feeling hungry or full.

Step 1: learn to examine your appestat

Check the appetite gauge beneath. I'm positive you can relate to those feelings.

Then, for the following week, keep a simple journal indicating your hunger or fullness throughout the day.

Once you've finished a few days of the journal, visit Step 2 and learn how to regulate your ingesting styles for satiety, weight reduction, and weight control.

Appetite Gauge

You're absolutely crammed! You're so complete you sense nauseous. This in all likelihood takes place after a banquet, including Thanksgiving, or after a binge.

You're uncomfortably complete. You experience bloated. This may arise after an eating place meal wherein you consume an appetizer, dinner, and dessert all within 30-40 minutes.

You're perfectly relaxed. Your experience satisfaction. this sense normally follows a wholesome, balanced meal. You can find a moderate longing for candy with this sensation, but it will leave within 5-10 minutes if left on its own.

You're slightly uncomfortable. You're simply starting to experience hungry. This normally sets into a few hours after a balanced meal. This sense needs to be a purple flag to find a meal or snack that includes protein, carbs, and fats as soon as viable.

You're very uncomfortable, and experience susceptible and lightheaded. You're not able to concentrate. This kind of hunger usually units in if you've skipped a meal, or if you've no longer eaten any protein all day lengthy

If that is a frequent prevalence, make sure to preserve a wholesome snack — along with almonds or a string cheese — available always!

Use your appestat to manipulate your hunger

If you've discovered that you're on the whole rating a 4 or 5 at the appestat that means you're regularly feeling too full, attempt these strategies:

Devour extra slowly. Goal to bite each bite of meals 10-15 times, and positioned your fork down in between bites.

Wait 10 minutes until you go back for 2nd helpings.

Divide your meals into servings that are eaten two hours apart.

If you discover which you're always rating a one or two, that means you're continually hungry, try these techniques:

Don't allow more than 3 hours to pass with the aid of without eating a meal or a snack.

Continually encompass a protein, carb, and fat in your meal or snack.

Make certain which you're ingesting ample calories and that those calories are spread evenly all through the day. you may want to bulk up your breakfast meal and let the calories taper because the day goes on.

If you locate that you're always rating a three that means you're quite glad most of the day, congratulations! You're probably consuming a balanced weight loss plan, with 4 to six mini-meals and snacks during the day. Keep up the good work.

CHAPTER TWO

WHY BURNING FAT IS BETTER THAN LOOSING WEIGHT

Do you need to shed pounds?

If you spoke back sure, you're incorrect. Nicely, no longer incorrect genuinely, however, what you're simply looking to do is lose fats. Each person can shed pounds. You simply don't eat. You may shed pounds; regrettably, the burden you lose can be both muscle and fats.

The goal of a hit weight reduction is to hold as plenty muscles as viable, or likely even advantage some, while at the equal time lose as plenty body fat as possible. Your body fat is a key indicator of your achievement, not the dimensions. In truth, stay offs the scale.

Muscle is critical in your achievement for dropping fats. Muscle groups have those little fats burning powerhouses referred to as mitochondria. Mitochondria are mobile power vegetation that can be liable for the production of strength. It's inside the mitochondria that fat is metabolized. There's a fantastic correlation between the amount of muscle you have got and the wide variety of mitochondria. And it stands to purpose that the extra mitochondria you've got the more the capability to burn fat.

Get extra Mitochondria

How do you get greater of those little cell powerhouses? You want to be giving your body a motive to create more of them. You do that by means of acting high-intensity exercising. HIIT schooling is just one of these methods. Weight training is any other. by developing a massive call for electricity up and above what your frame can already produce, your body is forced to create new mitochondria on the way to be prepared for the subsequent time your muscle tissue call on that wanted more electricity.

The extraordinary factor about muscle and mitochondria is that they are lively tissue. Unlike fat, they want consistent strength to hold themselves – strength like fatty acids. What does this mean? It means that your body might be burning fats at all times of the day – even while you're slumbering. Sure, its miles possible to burn fat for your sleep, and that are how.

Don't fear approximately Your Weight

Telling human beings to ignore their weight is a completely common theme for us, and for the appropriate motive. Too generally successful dieting is sabotaged because of a meaningless variety on a scale. A scale does nothing aside from the pressure of gravity for your body. Why ought to this be counted at all? It may let you know if your clothes healthy higher, it couldn't tell you if your body fat percent has modified, and it truly received tell you which you're looking any better.

Whilst you start a weight-reduction plan, it is vital which you music your progress the usage of strategies aside from the size. You need progress measuring gear that might be going to tune fat loss – no longer weight loss. body fat calipers, tape measures, photos, garments sizes, and those are feedback are all going to be extra useful for you. Don't worry about your weight – even supposing it goes up. If you're searching better, your weight doesn't depend.

Hold Muscle at the same time as dropping fats.

Humans generally tend to sabotage their diets by eating too few meals and too few nutrients ensuing in muscle loss. Once you start dropping muscle, you're combating an uphill struggle to lose fats. That is one of the principal motives why diets fail, simply in the back of meal addiction.

To prevent muscle loss, make sure you are following these simple pointers:

• Get insufficient calories to your body length and interest degree.

• ensure those energies are nutrient-dense via having them come from end result, veggies, meats, legumes, tubers, dairy, and whole grains.

• Intention for calories inside the 10-12 instances your frame weight variety.

• try to get in 1 gram of protein in keeping with pound of lean frame weight, and divide that frivolously amongst 5 meals.

• eat enough carbohydrates to support your interest level. You can start at a hundred and fifty grams and adjust from there.

• Fill the rest of your calories with fats – wholesome fat and EFAs (critical fatty acids).

• make certain you exercising and give your muscle groups a cause to preserve themselves. if you don't work out, your frame goes to shed that unneeded muscle. Force your frame to maintain it and even grow it by giving it consistent stimulation.

Comply with these hints and you may attain your authentic intention of no longer simply losing weight, however dropping that unwanted fat, and maintaining your beautiful muscle.

CHAPTER THREE

WHAT TO EAT OR AVOID EVERYDAY

Ingredients to perk you up:

Grapefruit

The smell of citrus culmination—like grapefruit—makes the frame more alert, consistent with the countrywide Sleep foundation. Not most effective will it assist wake you up, however, the scent of the citrus fruit also can reason your body to produce the happiness hormone, serotonin. Did we point out it is full of immunity-boosting diet c and waist-whittling outcomes? In fact, a have a look published within the magazine   Metabolism determined that consuming half of a grapefruit earlier than food may additionally help lessen viscerally (belly) fats and lower cholesterol levels.

Kale

Kale is filled with nutrients and minerals, making it the right addition to omelets or smoothies. It's a hearty supply of iron, which performs no small role in perking you up. Low iron stages can cause anemia that frequently results in fatigue and sluggishness.

Comprise greater kale in your weight loss plan with those 15+ exceptional wholesome Kale Recipes.

Eggs

Aside from being filled with choline, eggs have a B-diet that enhances brain and power characteristics and unsaturated fats, which keep you sharp and alert. Plus, eggs are full of protein! And not like many carbohydrates, protein is metabolized slowly, providing you with power that lasts during the day without weighing you down.

Foods to assist the stress:

Grape Juice

Does pressure have you ever in a daze? There are a growing number of research findings that recommend grape juice just is probably the treatment. In fact, a university of Leeds examines located that eating 12 each day oz. of grape juice could have long-lasting fine results on reminiscence and general performance for careworn-out people.

Avocado

While we are careworn, we regularly look for consolation

within the incorrect locations (like a bag of potato chips), which is why avocados are the pleasant stored anti-stress mystery. according to analyze posted within the vitamins magazine, consuming just one-half of avocado may prevent pointless snacking. The first rate-fruit is satiating and helps alter blood sugar—a combo that'll keep you out of the vending device, even in times of pressure!

Ingredients for when you're certainly hungry:

Greek Yogurt

When eleven: 45 A.M. hits and ghrelin (the hunger-inducing hormone) takes over, you do not need to absolutely sabotage your diet or your temper. One 6 ounce container of nonfat Greek yogurt is just one hundred calories and includes 17 grams of starvation-busting protein. Now, this not to say is packed to the brim with probiotics, which create a healthy intestine and enhance your immune system.

Apples

Apples contain energy-rich carbohydrates, sluggish-digesting fiber, and fructose, which is a herbal sugar that offers you the raise you need to make it thru your morning assembly as it digests slowly through the frame.

Almonds

Whether you reach for uncooked almonds or almond butter, the potent nuts boast coronary heart-healthful fat, flat belly fiber, and satiating protein. Better but, they are full of magnesium, which facilitates conversation sugar into power. This killer combination gives sustained strength without the submit-meal crash.

Foods that make you experience sleepy:

Cow's Milk

Despite the fact that cow's milk may be a part of a balanced weight-reduction plan, it is able to have negative outcomes to your electricity degrees. While we digest food, intestine hormones referred to as enterogastrones are released, which have an effect on blood float? Due to the fact dairy is not always digested without difficulty (especially whilst large amounts are ingested), plenty of blood is wanted to aid within the system, leaving less blood for the rest of the frame. This loss of blood can purpose lethargy.

Peanut Butter

Ever surprise why you get a bit sleepy after you devour a peanut butter sandwich? The satiating unfold consists of the amino acid tryptophan, which makes us worn-out. However, that doesn't mean you have to forgo the stuff altogether. Simply make certain to preserve it to one serving and pair it with electricity-boosting super foods to overcome the food coma.

French Fries

At the same time as a serving of carbs is right each now and again, having to a lot of them— like too much French fries—can motive blood sugar spikes and dips that result in sluggishness and mind fog.

THE END